Aerobics

The Invisible Advantage

By

Ronald Portal

AuthorHouse™
1663 Liberty Drive
Bloomington, IN 47403
www.authorhouse.com
Phone: 1 (800) 839-8640

Published by AuthorHouse 02/11/2020

ISBN: 978-1-4033-3515-9 (sc)

Print information available on the last page.

PROLOGUE

THE BIG CHOLESTEROL MIX UP

The Physical: Because excessive cholesterol surrounds hardening of the arteries it is wrongly assumed to be the cause. Read why an accelerated resting pulse rate is to blame and not cholesterol. We are being most influenced by the resting pulse rate a state we are in most of our lives. C-Reactive Protein measures inflammation in the arterial system. A weak arterial system means that the resting pulse rate must beat more often in order to supply the required blood. Because of the "Action Reaction Law" over a life time millions of extra beats cause damaging inflammation. Inflammation reduces arterial flexibility (hardening of the arteries). It is the arteries flexible activity that most prevents the buildup of excessive cholesterol. Cholesterol a substance we can't live without has received universal blame. Hard to believe but the accelerated resting pulse rate is the true villain. Exercise is the only way to lower the resting pulse rate. If we exercise for 30 minutes a day, during that period the pulse rate will be more rapid and intense but for the remaining 23 ½ hours because we strengthened the system the resting pulse rate will be slower and more efficient. For humans this life style should be consistent for a life time beginning during adolescence if not before. This game changer in priorities from diet to exercise provides the true foundation for life time prevention.

ACKNOWLEDGMENTS

In great appreciation for Erna Holyer's writing class.
A big thanks for all the guidance and support from
Erna and all my fellow students, especially Dave Self,
Lois Maggio, and Dale Tibbils.

About the Book

Arterial disease is the most serious health problem in the modern world. Isn't it curious, that with all this talk about including exercise in our life style, nowhere is there an explanation of how aerobic exercise prevents the buildup of cholesterol and hardening of the arteries? Many books describe the improved arterial profile resulting from aerobics. Extensive research has made it clear that exercise is extremely beneficial. Unfortunately, the actual cause-and-effect chain has not been understood.

In this book the information unfolds by way of a conversation between three human entities, The Mental, The Physical, and The Emotional. Revealed through their discussion are the reasons why a lack of aerobic exercise is to blame for hardening of the arteries, the development of excessive cholesterol on the inside walls of arteries, and weak collateral circulation.

As a physical educator, the author spent thirty-seven years teaching the aerobic preventive approach to arterial difficulties. He says, "We are talking about a muscle system that has been weakened by the inactivity of modern technology." This will be the first published explanation of how aerobics actually influences the inside diameter of arteries.

The projected readership will be physical educators, the medical community, athletes, and everyone possessing arteries. This fresh approach has no rival and represents a genuine advance in the prevention of arterial disease. We are not what we eat, but rather we are what we do.

TABLE OF CONTENTS

CHAPTER ONE

FACTS AND THEORIES

In which the three Voices, "Mental," "Emotional," and "Physical" that are part of all of us introduce the importance of a lower resting pulse rate and the need for aerobic exercise when we talk about reducing artery disease.

The Emotional: "You guys always end up arguing about which of you is more important and I always feel left out."

The Physical: "Well, behavior is a pretty big deal and my all-important muscle is responsible for every bit of it."

The Mental: "Yes, but none of your muscle behavior occurs without direction from my brain."

The Emotional: "See, there you go. I thought we were supposed to work together."

The Physical: "Well, we do work together."

The Emotional: "I could make the argument that it's my feeling good that should be the ultimate goal."

The Mental: "Yes, and feeling good often depends on how well The Physical and I work together but we don't always agree."

The Emotional: "See, there it is, you've regulated my well-being to whatever you guys come up with. You both forget that I'm often a major influence on the ability of each of you to function."

The Mental: "OK, I agree, but no matter what, I'm the one in charge. I make all the decisions."

The Physical: "That's fine as long as the decisions are in our collective best interest, but sometimes they aren't."

The Mental: "Balony! When have I ever made a bad decision?"

The Physical: "For starters, I'm concerned about your warped approach to arterial disease, which is our greatest life-threatening challenge."

The Mental: "Are you talking about heart disease here?"

The Physical: "When you use the term, 'heart disease,' you localize the problem to the heart when in fact arterial difficulties can occur throughout the body."

The Mental: "Well, the experts have been calling it heart disease for almost a century."

The Emotional: "Listen, sometimes the experts are wrong. Don't forget it was the experts who once believed the earth was flat."

The Mental: "That's a ridiculous comparison."

The Physical: "It may not be ridiculous when we consider that the general population believes that diet is the most important factor when it comes to preventing heart disease, when the most important influence should really be aerobic exercise."

The Mental: "Well, in general, the medical community has determined that it is the build up of cholesterol on the inside walls of arteries, often called atherosclerosis or plaque, that causes arteriosclerosis, which is frequently referred to as hardening or thickening of the arterial wall."

The Emotional: "So, many people believe that diet is the most important factor because it's the best way to control cholesterol consumption."

The Physical: "Exactly. Cholesterol is misunderstood. It's really a lack of aerobic exercise that contributes most to arterial disease."

The Emotional: "I do hear exercise mentioned but usually in a supportive role and not as the primary factor as is the case with diet."

The Physical: "Exercise has a secondary status because just how aerobics retards the development of excessive cholesterol and arteriosclerosis hasn't been recognized."

The Emotional: "That's true. I've read the results of extensive research on exercise, and the experts always mention the importance of an exercise life-style, but there's never an explanation of exactly how aerobics changes the inside of the arterial system."

The Mental: "Physical, are you telling us that cholesterol doesn't cause hardening of the arteries?"

The Physical: "Yes, that's exactly what I'm saying."

The Mental: "Well if cholesterol isn't responsible for hardening of the arteries, then what is to blame?

The Physical: "It's a rapid resting pulse rate that causes arteriosclerosis."

The Mental: "Physical, you've got to be crazy to make such a claim. It's common knowledge that cholesterol causes hardening of the arteries, excuse me, arteriosclerosis."

The Physical: "No, it isn't cholesterol, it's that overlooked resting pulse rate that's to blame. Aerobic exercise reduces an excessive resting pulse rate.

The Mental: "I've never heard that before. It sounds like a really off-the-wall idea. I'd rather rely on facts."

The Physical: "What facts are you talking about?"

The Mental: "Everyone knows that excessive accumulation of cholesterol on the inside wall of the artery causes hardening of the arteries."

The Physical: "It's true that arteriosclerosis or hardening of the arteries is always accompanied by excessive amounts of cholesterol 'atherosclerosis', but to assume that the cholesterol is the cause of the thickening of the arterial wall is pure theory."

The Mental: "It seems to me that all that consistency strongly supports the theory.

The Physical: "No matter how consistent the appearance, it's only an unverified theory because there's no explanation of how all that cholesterol actually causes the hardening and thickening of the arterial wall."

The Mental: "Then the experts are wrong?"

The Physical: "The experts have arrived at a perfectly reasonable conclusion. However, it's not an explanation, it's only an assumption."

The Emotional: "What about my stress? I thought it was a fact that my stress level contributes to heart disease."

The Physical: "You're right, research demonstrates that people with arterial problems often show high stress."

The Emotional: "Well then, doesn't that kind of research consistency make it a fact?"

The Physical: "As with cholesterol, the overwhelming connection between stress levels and heart disease isn't ignored by the experts. There's a strong correlation. It would only be fact if the actual effect of stress on the arterial system could be explained."

The Mental: "So, Physical, are you saying that your resting pulse rate idea is really the one we should be focusing on?"

The Physical: "Yes, aerobic exercise strengthens arterial muscle which lowers the resting pulse rate's pace. It's not only the most logical explanation, but it's the only one that's accompanied by a description of cause and effect."

The Mental: "Now that you mention it, I must agree. We're constantly being told that exercise is good for us without ever hearing why."

The Emotional: "That's interesting, I have noticed that a sedentary life-style, or more specifically a lack of aerobic exercise, is always presented as one of the health risk factors."

The Physical: "Yes, and extensive research involving aerobic exercise has demonstrated its considerable benefits for good health."

The Emotional: "Well, that all sounds pretty factual. Why haven't the effects of aerobics been told to us?"

The Physical: "Prior to this conversation, the influence of aerobics on the arteries has never been explained. This has the effects of exercise as correlated but not proven."

The Mental: "You've got to be off-base. Don't you realize that your going against a long established majority opinion?"

The Physical: "Listen, Mental, don't you find it curious that in spite of all the supporting evidence, there has never been an explanation of how aerobics reduces hardening of the artery walls and build-up of cholesterol, the two conditions that most narrow the inside diameter of the artery?"

The Mental: "That does seem strange. Why is that?"

The Physical: "It simply hasn't been understood."

The Emotional: "Are you saying that exercise is the ultimate form of prevention when so many other sources are claiming prevention comes from diet, drugs, herbs, acupuncture, meditation, psychotherapy and other treatments?"

The Physical: "Each of those approaches might play a comparatively small role and might make a contribution to prevention. However, in terms of influence, compared with aerobic exercise, they all have insignificant effects. Before all else we are talking about a muscle system that has been allowed to become weak. This is why the exercise approach demands the initial focus."

The Emotional: "It's true. Second to diet, I always hear exercise mentioned in relationship to prevention and treatment of heart disease. It never occurred to me that I haven't seen or heard an explanation of that relationship."

The Physical: "Only two positive conditions have been identified as the results of doing aerobic exercise. First, aerobics are said to be the best way to create good cholesterol, but with no follow-up about how this prevents cholesterol from building up on the inside walls of the arteries. Second, aerobics raises the heart rate, and here again the benefits of an elevated heart rate aren't described."

The Mental: "And I suppose you're going to explain all these aerobic benefits?"

The Physical: "Of course. How else can I help you make the proper decisions about our behavior?"

The Mental: "Very funny."

The Physical: "During the twentieth century, Many arterial hypotheses were developed. Every conceivable medicine, food, and behavior was thought to be either the cause of heart disease or its savior. I'm convinced that aerobic exercise will emerge as the single most effective regimen when it comes to both prevention and treatment."

The Mental: "I'm not convinced. Fortunately we have my all-important brain to help us figure out these problems."

The Physical: "Actually it's your brain that has contributed most to the problems we're having."

CHAPTER TWO

TECHNOLOGY'S REDUCTION OF ACTIVITY

In which Technology, Mental's creature, gets a lot of blame.

The Mental: "How can you say that it's my brain's fault?"

The Physical: "It's the modern technology that your brain helped to develop that has dramatically reduced human physical behavior all of which is the result of my muscle performance."

The Mental: "What do you mean by that?"

The Physical: "Can you think of a body movement that doesn't involve muscle?"

The Mental: "OK, but listen, Physical, because of all my marvelous technology, your muscle gets to kick back and take it easy."

The Emotional: "It's true, many living in modern societies are enjoying doing less."

The Physical: "That's the problem, Mental. Prior to your invention of the steam engine, humans had much more active lives. Your modern technology has caused the general population to become very sedentary. Muscle that doesn't get used degenerates quickly. The heart and arteries are the most important muscle system suffering from this change."

The Emotional: "Arteries have muscle?"

The Physical: "Everyone understands that the heart is muscle, but not many people know that part of the walls of all arteries is muscle too. That's why I like to refer to it as our muscular arterial system, heart and arteries."

The Emotional: "Mental, all of your technological progress during the 20th century has really kicked my stress level up. Unexpected life change is my greatest nemesis."

The Mental: "Don't be such a baby. Change is a normal and ongoing process."

The Emotional: "Yes, but because of your modern technology more change has occurred during the past century than during all the human time preceding it. I realize that change is continuous, but so much change in such a short period of time is the major source of my stress."

The Mental: "It's true. My third technological shock, the steam engine, has accelerated beneficial change for all humankind."

The Emotional: "Increasing my stress level is not beneficial."

The Mental: "You had better get used to it. My technology has always increased the rate of change. We'll get to your stress business later. I want to hear more about The Physical's exercise stuff."

The Physical: "You're right. Most of your new technology is positive, but it's meant a tremendous reduction in physical activity, every bit of which is expressed through my muscle."

The Mental: "Isn't that good?"

The Physical: "No, because it violates the 'Use it or lose it' law that regulates all muscle."

CHAPTER THREE

MUSCLE AND TECHNOLOGY

In which we are introduced to the "Use it or lose it" law and Mental's theory about three technological shocks.

The Mental: "Use it or lose it law, what's that?"

The Physical: "I believe this is true for all animal functions, but we know that when muscle is used it becomes stronger and more efficient and when muscle isn't used it begins to atrophy and degenerate."

The Mental: "How do you know this? Is it just another one of your goofy theories?"

The Physical: "No, the 'Use it or lose it' law is fact. Whenever skeletal muscle is exposed to weight resistant training programs, it becomes measurably larger and stronger."

The Emotional: "What happens if muscle isn't used?"

The Physical: "There once was a physical education teacher who, in order to make this point, brought a football player into his class. A five week old cast had just been removed from the player's broken leg. The class could clearly see that the leg that had been inhibited by the cast was much smaller than the leg that hadn't."

The Emotional: "I can believe that. I've often noticed while watching tennis matches that the racquet arms of many players are larger than the non-racquet arms."

The Mental: "OK, I understand that, but does it mean that people who exercise will never lose muscle?"

The Physical: "No, of course not. Some time between the age of fifteen and twenty-five the human animal becomes physically mature. After that muscles, and related systems, begin a long slow period of degeneration. Exercise is simply the most effective way of postponing or slowing that degeneration. There is no fountain of youth."

The Mental: "You guys are trying to make my wonderful technology the villain for your theory. Listen, my brain has been kicking that stuff out forever."

The Emotional: "How do you know that?"

The Mental: "Human-made tools have been found that are much older than the earliest discovered human remains. Because of my brain and the resulting technology, humans have ascended to the top of the food chain and should be referred to as the technological animal. I can reasonably argue three technological shocks."

The Emotional: "What do you mean by shocks?"

The Mental: "I would like to let the word 'shock' represent the three most important and influential events in our human past."

The Emotional: "That's a mighty bold statement. The Physical and I are certainly aware of the third shock, the machine age, which began with the steam engine. What are the other two technological shocks?"

The Mental: "With my theory, the first shock was stick and stone technology. This shock was responsible for the greatest change of all. It forced the human animal to walk upright. Hands were so busy using 'sticks and stones' that they could no longer be used for locomotion."

The Physical: "That makes sense, but I'm mostly concerned about strenuous survival behavior, which was in no way reduced by your first shock as was the case with shock three."

The Mental: "My second shock was the great technological achievement of learning how to create and control fire. Humans, previously restricted to warmer regions, could migrate throughout the planet."

The Physical: "I agree here as well. Your second shock had a huge impact on humanity. It had to increase nomadism. When the 'Use it or lose it' law is applied, we can draw conclusions about why the legs are the largest muscle groups on the human frame."

The Mental: "You take your 'Use it or lose it' law too far."

The Physical: "Not at all. We can take the theory one step further. For many species, humans included, the males are bigger and stronger than the females. This is because the males have always engaged in a full range of motion."

The Emotional: "What do you mean by a full range of motion?"

The Physical: "Males ranged far and wide while females had to stay closer to home. The female range of motion has been inhibited by the birthing and nurturing responsibilities."

The Mental: "Well, anyway, those are the three technological shocks and my brain is responsible."

The Physical: "Listen Mental, you give too much credit to your brain. Other animals such as dolphins have more sophisticated nervous systems than humans. Dolphins don't have hands and it's hands that truly separate humans from the rest of the animal world."

The Mental: "Are you now saying that your hands are more important than my brain?"

The Physical: "I was glad to hear you mention that hands participated in your first technological shock. If, as you say, humans are the technological animal, then my all-important hands have been involved in every single bit of technology that has ever been developed."

The Mental: "You make a good case for body system interdependency, but my brain still rules."

The Physical: "Yes, but muscle is more important than you may realize. Muscle represents sixty to seventy percent of our total body mass. What often goes unnoticed is that the primary responsibility for all other systems is muscle function."

The Mental: "I find that hard to believe."

The Physical: "Hey, muscle is at the center of things. Bones support it, skin covers and protects it, the stomach prepares the fuel for it and, of all things, Mental, your brain spends over ninety-five percent of its time dealing with muscle activity."

The Mental: "Physical, you keep blaming arterial disease on my modern technology. Arterial disease has been on the scene for centuries. Sometime during the second half of the 20th century, the arteries of Egyptian mummies were examined. The arteries of these preserved individuals were found to possess large amounts of arteriosclerosis. Researchers have concluded that this disease has been around for a long time."

The Physical: "Yes, that's true, but only for the social elite of those times. The mummified individuals that researchers examined were at the top of their social order and were probably carried everywhere they went. Exercise, and especially aerobic exercise, was not a part of their living routine."

The Emotional: "I can believe that."

The Physical: "Those individuals were the very few exceptions and not representative of the general population. If we could have examined the arteries of people who were working on the pyramids, we would have discovered a very different arteriosclerosis profile. Mental, it's your modern technology that's caused the general population to become inactive."

The Mental: "Is all that muscle in trouble because it's not forced to be used as it once was?"

The Physical: "Yes, Mental, your technology reduces the activity level for all muscle."

CHAPTER FOUR

AEROBICS

Here the "Physical" talks about aerobic exercise and strengthening arterial muscle.

The Physical: "My theory really centers on the muscular arterial system, which includes the heart and arteries, and on the aerobic exercise that controls its strength."

The Mental: "Why is that system a big deal?

The Physical: "This muscle system is the most important, not just because it must provide the entire body with blood, but because it's the most threatened. It's a system that starts up long before birth, frequently continues for a short time after death and, of course, is at work for a lifetime in between."

The Mental: "How does the arterial muscle perform?"

The Physical: "The arterial muscle of the heart and arteries pumps, expands, contracts, squeezes, and drives the blood toward its destination. Mental, prior to your 20th century technology, aerobic exercise, which is the only way arterial muscle can be strengthened, was a natural and consistent result of most human activity."

The Mental: "What do you mean by aerobic exercise?"

The Physical: "All animals, including humans, have a wide range of activity levels. The range is from complete calm, rest, or sleep, to extended periods of activity using large portions of skeletal muscle. This accelerated activity or exercise is referred to as aerobic."

The Emotional: "How do we know if we have had an aerobic experience?"

The Physical: "Aerobic exercise is any activity that lasts 20 to 30 minutes or longer. The three by-products of aerobics are increased heart or pulse rate, oxygen debt or shortness of breath, and perspiration."

The Emotional: "Some humans claim that they never sweat."

The Physical: "That may be true if we call heavy, runny, drippy perspiration 'sweat'. However, a slightly moistened skin is also a sign of perspiration, and happens to everyone. This light perspiration level is an aerobic message that the beginner shouldn't ignore. As strength improves, more effort will be required in order to produce the same amount of perspiration."

The Mental: "So why are aerobics so important?"

The Physical: "Aerobics, which occurred naturally prior to your steam engine, are the only way to exercise arterial muscle."

The Mental: "What's that got to do with your resting pulse rate theory?"

The Physical: "My theory says that the absence of aerobic exercise causes the arterial system to become weaker. The 'Use it or lose it' law is being violated. As the arterial system gets weaker it must beat more often in order to distribute the same volume of blood. The extra beats of the increased resting pulse rate cause damage to the arteries, usually where they fork."

The Mental: "How can you theorize that your aerobic exercise occurred naturally before my third shock?"

The Physical: "Before your modern technology, the feeding pattern was responsible for most of human activity. Throughout the last ten thousand years agriculture without machines made aerobic activity necessary."

The Mental: "That's a relatively short period of time. What about before that?"

The Physical: "My theory concludes that prior to that, nomadism, hunting and gathering, and survival in general required constant aerobic exercise. Your third shock has eliminated, for most of us, our participation in the feeding pattern and the extensive physical activity it required."

The Mental: "Yes, relieving modern humans of their previously demanding feeding pattern responsibilities has been one of my greatest, if somewhat overlooked, achievements.

The Emotional: "Listen, Mental, all forms of life spend most of their thought and activity getting food. Because of your technology, the Physical is alarmed about the huge drop in human physical activity. My big concern is social disruption. Powerful, interdependent survival responsibilities required by the feeding pattern, the ones that are most responsible for the social glue, are lost forever."

The Mental: "Emotional, you're trying to change the subject. Let's stay with the physical thing. Physical, the inactivity of today's modern world makes it difficult to envision what you describe. Was there really that much aerobic activity?"

The Physical: "For those who can't imagine pre-machine activity, let me make a case for human eyebrows. Eyebrows are important clues to our human aerobic past."

The Mental: "Eyebrows? Now you've really lost it."

The Physical: "We all have eyebrows. This, Mental, is because your brain must be kept cool. During aerobic exercise, the head perspires to cool us more profusely than the rest of the body. The forehead is especially active. Eyebrows guide the salty sweat away from the eyes so that our vision will not be impaired during aerobic activities."

The Mental: "So my technology is responsible for this gigantic change in physical behavior. Physical, you are a Luddite."

The Emotional: "What's a Luddite?"

The Mental: "A Luddite is someone who opposes technology and all its change."

The Physical: "I don't oppose technology. Like you, I believe that humans are the technological animal. But I also believe that it's important for humans to recognize that major changes in long-standing behaviors may have negative influences on their health. When the problem is understood, proper adaptations can be applied."

The Emotional: "That means, Mental, that you have a better chance to make good decisions about our collective well-being."

The Mental: "Oh Emotional, just butt out."

The Physical: "Before your third shock, humans were running, jumping, climbing, active animals. Mental, in your modern world, a human could go for an entire lifetime without drawing a deep breath. Because it requires a great deal of effort, aerobics was one of the first behaviors that you figured out how to eliminate with your third shock."

The Mental: "Physical, give me an example of an adaptation to your arterial disease problem."

The Physical: "Reasonable humans, realizing that one out of two people will experience arterial disease, and understanding that eliminating natural aerobic behavior is the main cause of the problem, will artificially program aerobic exercise into their life style."

The Emotional: "That sounds logical."

The Physical: "By doing this, they will be playing the highest possible percentages when it comes to extending active, enjoyable life."

The Emotional: "I am not a Luddite either and I fully recognize the importance of humankind's unalterable relationship with technology. I can also identify some negative social aspects of the move away from the feeding pattern."

The Mental: "You sure are persistent."

The Emotional: "I am especially interested in the degeneration of the family structure that occurred during the 20th century. It has had a negative influence on society in general and it's major source of stress for me."

The Mental: "Hey! let's stay on track here. Emotional, we can get to your social stuff later. I need to hear more about arterial disease and The Physical's resting pulse rate theory."

CHAPTER FIVE

ARTERIAL DISEASE

In which the three arterial disease culprits are
identified.

The Mental: "Physical, you keep talking about
aerobic exercise and heart disease. It seems to me that
during the 20th century, much greater emphasis was
placed on proper diet than there was placed on
exercise. One of the major health statements for the
past century was, 'You are what you eat.'"

The Physical: "That's correct. 'You are what you
eat' may well be the health statement for the 20th
century. That's because we have come to believe,
wrongly, that cholesterol causes arteriosclerosis, which
is hardening of the arteries."

The Mental: "That's the general consensus."

The Physical: "This thick and hardened condition,
along with excessive cholesterol build-up on the inside
walls of the arteries, are the two reasons that the inside
diameters of arteries become narrowed. Weak
collateral circulation, which refers to the number of
available arteries that are functioning, is the third
arterial disease partner."

The Emotional: "So excessive hardening of the
arteries, the build-up of excessive cholesterol, and
weak collateral circulation are the three components of

arterial disease? There must be other things that can go wrong."

The Physical: "Yes, but causes beyond the big three are statistically insignificant. These are the three conditions that work together to form arterial disease and almost never do we find one without the presence of the other two."

The Mental: "And aerobics is the answer to all three of these problems? Come on."

The Physical: "I will demonstrate that all three of these conditions are reduced or postponed more by aerobic exercise than any other treatment or combination of treatments."

The Mental: "What about the diet angle?

The Physical: "Arterial disease was responsible for more deaths during the 20th century than all other causes combined. We mostly blame cholesterol and we've come to believe that the best way to control cholesterol levels is through our diet. Therefore, 'We are what we eat.'"

The Emotional: "Makes sense to me."

The Physical: "We are beginning the 21st century believing that when it comes to preventing arterial disease, diet should be the most important consideration, with exercise and drugs playing support roles."

The Mental: "Then you agree and I'm right."

The Physical: "No, I disagree, and you are wrong. The 20th century produced some major misconceptions about this disease."

The Mental: "Give me some examples."

The Physical: "Well to start with, we use the wrong name. Heart disease is a 20th century term. In the 21st century it will be referred to as arterial disease, which of course it is."

The Mental: "What's the difference?"

The Physical: "During the 20th century and up to the present, heart disease and stroke were incorrectly considered separate diseases, with separate statistics maintained for each."

The Emotional: "They sound different."

The Physical: "Heart attacks occur when the arteries to that muscle can no longer provide a blood supply. Here weak arterial muscle is less efficient and must beat more rapidly in order to meet the demand. Heart beats that are closer to the source are more damaging to the arteries, usually where they fork.

The Emotional: Why is that damage bad?"

The Physical: "That hardening, thickening, less flexible damaged area encourages the accumulation of cholesterol. These two conditions, working together, dangerously narrow the inside diameter of arteries. Blockage of arteries that supply the heart muscle itself often occurs and we call it a 'heart attack,'

The Mental: "What about stroke?"

The Physical: "Stroke occurs, Mental, when the arteries that supply your brain fail to provide an adequate supply of blood to it. There are two major kinds of stroke: ischemic and hemorrhagic. About 80 percent of strokes are ischemic. Ischemic stroke is a cutoff of blood due to blockage. Sometimes this blockage is the result of arteriosclerosis but more often because of a withering collateral circulation."

The Emotional: "What happens with hemorrhagic stroke?"

The Physical: "Hemorrhagic stroke is bleeding in the brain from a ruptured artery or vein and is attributed to high blood pressure or physical injury.

Ischemic and hemorrhagic stroke both result in an interruption in the delivery of blood and along with heart attack represent an inefficient supply system. Heart attack and stroke are both the result of "arterial disease".

The Emotional: "The current ranking of killers is: heart disease number one, cancer number two, and stroke number three. Are you saying that heart attack and stroke should be in a common category referred to as arterial disease?"

The Physical: "Exactly. Heart attack and stroke are both the result of arterial deficiency."

The Emotional: "Well what about hypertension?"

The Physical: "Of course you're right. Irregular blood pressure, as hypertension is often referred to, is a message about inefficient arterial function. Although often treated separately, it's clearly a symptom of arterial disease."

The Mental: "You said it was a degenerative disease. Doesn't that make it natural?"

The Physical: "Yes, this degenerative disease can be considered a natural event when it occurs at ages seventy, eighty, and above. However, in your hi-tech, mechanical world, this isn't the case. Arterial disease is occurring in significant numbers of people who are in their thirties, forties, and fifties."

The Emotional: "These are age groups, that by other standards reflect the human animal's 'prime of life'."

The Physical: "It's because the muscular arterial system never gets used that it becomes weak and fails prematurely. If we can adapt, the health statement for the 21st century will be 'You are what you do'."

The Emotional: "So arterial disease has three parts?"

The Physical: "Yes. Excessive cholesterol, excessive hardening of the arteries, and excessively weak collateral circulation."

The Emotional: "Why do you use the words excessive and excessively?"

The Physical: "It's because these three degenerative conditions always exist. The trick is preventing them from becoming excessive."

The Emotional: "Well let's talk about cholesterol."

CHAPTER SIX

CHOLESTEROL

Why something so necessary is so misunderstood.

The Mental: "It seems to me that all available information strongly connects excessive cholesterol to improper diet. Isn't it true that most food containers have labels listing cholesterol content and don't products brag when cholesterol contents are low?"

The Physical: "Yes, it's true, and the connection between diet and excessive cholesterol has been incorrectly over-emphasized. We aren't sure of all the reasons we have cholesterol but we know that it plays an important role in transporting fuel to individual cells and has some hormonal responsibilities. All humans have cholesterol, we can't live with out it, most foods contain it, and should the body run short, it can produce its own in the liver."

The Emotional: "If cholesterol is such an important item, how come it has such a dirty name?"

The Physical: "It's because cholesterol is somewhat misunderstood. Cholesterol is present in two forms. When it's in the blood fluid, it's called serum cholesterol. It's also in a more waxy solid form that builds up on the inside of the arterial wall and is referred to as atherosclerosis or sometimes called plaque. It is this second form that tends to accumulate on the inner lining and begins to narrow the inside diameter of the artery. It's one of two reasons that cholesterol has acquired a bad name."

The Mental: "Earlier you used the word excessive. Does this plaque always exists?"

The Physical: "A thin layer of cholesterol is normal, probably a reserve. It's when this layer becomes extreme and the build-up excessive that arteries begin to develop reduced inside dimensions."

The Mental: "Well, what's this business about good cholesterol and bad cholesterol?"

The Physical: "Two quality levels of cholesterol have been identified. They are 'good' cholesterol or high density lipoprotein, HDL, and 'bad' cholesterol or low density lipoprotein, LDL. HDL are tiny molecules that don't take up much room and are extremely efficient at performing cholesterol's responsibilities. LDL are large molecules consuming valuable space inside the artery, that are very weak at performing cholesterol's duties."

The Mental: "Do aerobics play a role here?"

The Physical: "Yes, this is the single area in which the experts have identified cause and effect. Aerobic exercise is the most effective way to create high density lipoprotein, HDL, the good cholesterol."

The Emotional: "You make it sound so simple. With the athlete, all the cells with cholesterol layers are lean, mean, and certainly more efficient."

The Physical: "Yes, and the larger LDL, of a sedentary individual, takes up valuable space and is less effective at performing its responsibilities."

The Mental: Isn't lipoprotein quality determined by testing serum cholesterol?"

The Emotional: "What do you mean by serum cholesterol testing?"

The Physical: "That's testing the amount and quality of cholesterol contained within the blood fluid."

The Mental: "Physical, what about the more solid form that builds up on the inside of the artery wall, that you called atherosclerosis or plaque?"

The Physical: "Yes, that's the more dangerous form because as it accumulates it narrows the inside diameter of the artery. Most current testing reveals serum cholesterol content, but doesn't expose the amount of atherosclerosis that has built up on the inner wall of arteries, which is the most important condition."

The Mental: "Well how does your aerobic exercise prevent the cholesterol from building up on the inside wall of the artery?"

CHAPTER SEVEN

AEROBICS AND CHOLESTEROL

How to prevent the build up of cholesterol on the inner lining of arteries.

The Mental: "Well, that cholesterol form, that plaque that builds up on the inside of the arterial wall, is a fatty substance. It still makes sense that diet is the most important factor when it comes to the accumulation of cholesterol or that plaque. What's the big deal about your aerobic exercise?"

The Physical: "Aerobics, which had been occurring naturally for all pre-modern technological time, creates a greater demand for oxygen.

The Mental: "How does this demand for oxygen influence the two cholesterols? The fluid form that's serum cholesterol and the solid form that builds up on the inner wall of the artery and becomes atherosclerosis?"

The Physical: "Because of the extensive testing conducted on serum cholesterol it's known that exercise creates good cholesterol."

The Mental: "You said earlier that it was the atherosclerosis building up on the inside of the artery wall that was most important and seldom tested."

The Physical: "Yes, testing for excessive deposited cholesterol or for hardening of the arteries, is more complicated and is generally not part of a routine checkup."

The Mental: "Well then, how does aerobics' increased demand for oxygen influence atherosclerosis?"

The Physical: "This demand triggers two important changes in the arterial system. First, the heart must beat faster in order to accommodate this increased demand for oxygen. Second, and most important for our purposes, the artery has the capacity to, and does, expand in order to help accommodate the larger and more rapidly flowing supply of blood. When the aerobic activity is complete, the artery will shrink back to its resting pulse rate diameter."

The Mental: "That makes sense, but why is that expansion and contraction important?"

The Physical: "It's that expansion and contraction, with the resulting stretching and disturbance to the inner wall of the artery, that inhibits the build-up of excessive cholesterol. Not only is there a normal disturbance to the inside wall of the artery, but at the same time, blood is moving through the system with a great deal more force and helps to flush cholesterol out."

The Emotional: "Sounds like a cleansing action to me.

The Physical: "These natural agitations, the stretching and disturbance to the inner wall of the artery caused by expansion and contraction and the flushing behavior of the increased flow, can only be created by aerobic exercise. It's those important aerobic changes within the arterial system that inhibits the buildup of excessive cholesterol on the inner walls of the arteries."

The Emotional: "So in the machine-age society, an individual may go for long periods of time, or all of life without drawing a deep breath. This lack of aerobics means that the arteries never get expanded and the inner walls never gets disturbed.

The Physical: "Yes, this modern world behavioral change, from active to inactive, encourages the buildup of excessive cholesterol on the inner wall of the artery. The build-up narrows the inside diameter of the artery. This dramatically reduces arterial efficiency and creates high potential for arterial occlusion, which means getting plugged up."

The Mental: "What about all this cholesterol testing? It seems like a lot of humans are using these tests to measure their arterial health."

The Physical: "Today, testing blood serum for cholesterol quantity and quality are standard procedures during most physical examinations. These tests are clues, but don't tell us how much cholesterol has built up on the inside walls of the arteries, which is the most important concern. It's possible that the cholesterol level in the blood serum is genetically programmed."

The Mental: "What makes you think it's genetic?"

The Physical: "Often people complain that they are aerobic and careful with their diet and still have a high cholesterol count. Because of the aerobic exercise, and the resulting expansion and contraction of the artery, those individuals have created a thin and healthy layer of cholesterol on the inner wall of the artery regardless of their serum test results."

The Emotional: "I frequently hear people say that they don't exercise or worry about their diet and yet have very low cholesterol test results."

The Physical: "Because there is no aerobic exercise, the arteries of these individuals never get disturbed and atherosclerosis is allowed to develop, a condition not revealed through current blood serum cholesterol testing.

The Mental: "Speaking of genetics, isn't it true that many people believe that this whole arterial disease business is in the genes and that humans really have very little control over it?"

The Physical: "It's true that genetics are important, but aerobic exercise still plays a major role. For an example, an acquaintance Frank was a runner and exercised everyday. He did so because there was a history of heart disease in his family. His father died at age forty and his mother at age forty-five both of heart attacks. Frank died of arterial disease at age sixty-two, and doctors agreed that his aerobic exercise had extended his life by ten to fifteen years."

The Mental: "Well, Physical, you've convinced me. When it comes to controlling excessive cholesterol, aerobic exercise is more important than diet."

The Physical: "Yes, Mental, it's important to understand that there is no diet that will disturb the inner walls of arteries. This can only be achieved with the aerobic exercise that had been occurring naturally until modern times."

The Mental: "You said earlier that arterial disease had three parts. Obviously, excessive atherosclerosis is one, so what are the other two?"

The Physical: "One is arteriosclerosis which is hardening of the arteries. The third and final part is 'collateral circulation,' which refers to the number of available arteries that are functioning."

The Emotional: "Well, tell us about arteriosclerosis."

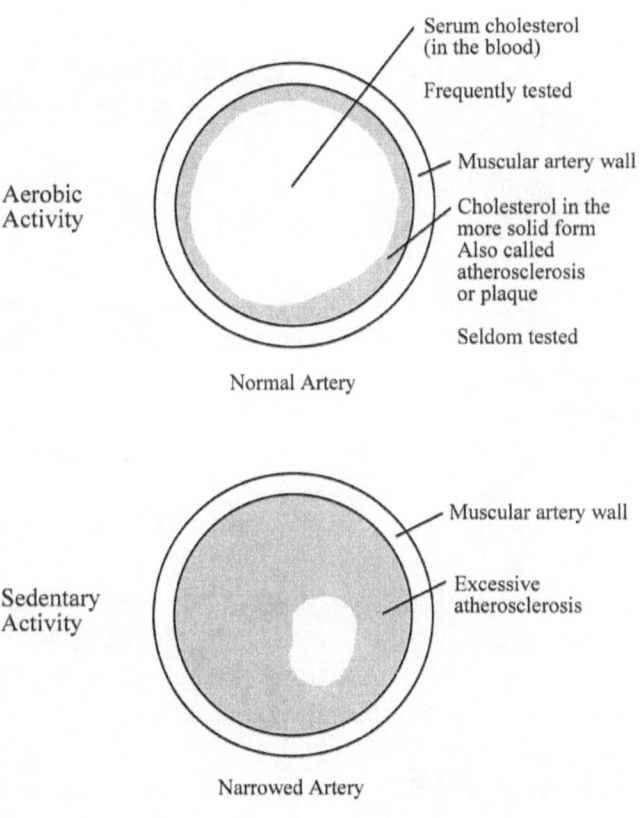

Aerobic
Activity

Serum cholesterol
(in the blood)

Frequently tested

Muscular artery wall

Cholesterol in the
more solid form
Also called
atherosclerosis
or plaque

Seldom tested

Normal Artery

Sedentary
Activity

Muscular artery wall

Excessive
atherosclerosis

Narrowed Artery

CHOLESTEROL

CHAPTER EIGHT

ARTERIOSCLEROSIS (HARDENING OF THE ARTERIES)

Why an elevated resting pulse rate is the culprit.
Numbers don't lie.

The Physical: "Arteriosclerosis is a fibrous, inflexible thickening of the arterial wall, often referred to as hardening of the arteries. This condition also causes a narrowing of the inside diameter of the artery. It's clearly the most misunderstood part of arterial disease."

The Mental: "What do you mean when you say it's misunderstood?"

The Physical: "For years, the experts have been telling us that excessive cholesterol or atherosclerosis causes arteriosclerosis. This is because arteriosclerosis is surrounded by exceptional amounts of atherosclerosis."

The Emotional: "Listen, I get confused. The words atherosclerosis and arteriosclerosis sound too much alike and I have trouble following the conversation. Why don't you just say that the places where hardening of the arteries occur are always surrounded by large amounts of cholesterol?"

The Physical: "OK, that sounds good. Anyhow, there's always a large buildup of cholesterol around the hardening of the arteries, which has made it easy to assume that it was the extra buildup of cholesterol that was damaging the arteries. In reality, it's the other way around. Hardening of the arteries contributes to the excessive buildup of cholesterol."

The Mental: "Well if it's not cholesterol, what is causing the damage to the arteries?"

The Physical: "It is the resting pulse rate that causes hardening or scarring of the arteries. This thickened condition known as arteriosclerosis may occur anywhere in the system but is most frequently found at the fork of an artery."

The Emotional: "Why is this hardened condition found most often where the arteries fork?"

The Physical: "Because the fork is directly in the path of the blood flow. If blood flowed evenly through our arteries, we wouldn't have a problem. But blood doesn't flow evenly through our arteries: it's pulsated. Just feel the pulse on your wrist to experience this phenomenon."

The Physical: "Its most likely behavioral heredity rather than genetic. Sisters and brothers being raised by inactive parents."

The Mental: "So what's the big deal?"

The Physical: "Every time the heart contracts it sends a spurt of blood into the artery. When this spurt comes to a fork, it strikes a blow. Half the spurt goes in one direction and half in the other. The blow struck represents damage, minute damage, but damage none the less. It's because damage most often occurs at the fork of the artery that multiple bypass surgeries are required. It's the resting pulse rate that must take center stage."

The Mental: "The resting pulse rate. I expected you to ramble on about the exercising pulse rate."

The Physical: "No, humans are exposed to the resting pulse rate for most of their lives. All night long, riding in their cars, in the work place, sitting in front of T.V.s and so forth. Because the arterial system is in a relaxed state most of the time, bodies are most influenced by the resting pulse rate."

The Emotional: "What about the popular stint procedure that widens the inside of arteries?"

The Physical: "Stints are effective for the short term; however, unlike aerobics, stints completely rob the artery of any existing flexibility potential."

The Emotional: "How about people who are really active?"

The Physical: "A marathon runner may run for two hours a day, but for the other twenty-two hours, he or she is in a resting state."

The Mental: "You're certainly not going to tell us that something as natural as the resting pulse rate is the main cause for humankind's number one killer? Heart beats begin months before birth, frequently extend for a short time after death, and continue for all the time in between. How can you blame hardening of the arteries on the resting pulse rate, something that can't possibly be avoided?"

The Physical: "It can't be avoided, but with aerobic exercise the resting pulse rate is dramatically reduced."

The Mental: "You know, Physical, that's not big news. I frequently hear medical people claim that aerobic exercise slows the heart rate."

The Physical: "Yes, research has confirmed that aerobics lowers the resting pulse rate, but the benefits of a lower resting pulse rate have never, until now, been explained."

The Emotional: "Well, what happens if there's no aerobic exercise?"

The Physical: "It's the 'Use it or lose it' law. When the muscular arterial system goes without exercise it becomes weaker. This means it must beat more often in order to distribute the blood with its life- sustaining nutrients and oxygen."

The Mental: "Why is a rise in the resting pulse rate important?"

The Physical: "The increase of a few extra beats in the average resting pulse rate will cause thousands of extra blows to be struck on the arterial forks each day. Because that resting pulse rate is responsible for excessive hardening of the arteries, it must be considered the most important body measurement.

The Mental: "Well then, What's the average resting pulse rate for humans?"

"The Physical: "Unfortunately, we will never know what the average resting pulse rate is for the human animal. Science has only been studying this measurement for about a hundred and fifty years, well inside the advent of your modern technology, and most of that within the 20th century."

The Mental: "Well, then, do we have an average or not?"

The Physical: "No, Mental, you haven't been listening. Your machine-age impact on our behavior has been so over- whelming that the currently accepted average resting pulse rate of seventy should be considered too high. Because aerobics was common behavior for all of pre-machine living, the average resting pulse rate was certainly much lower. However, it will never be known by how many beats."

The Mental: "What difference does it make if the pre- machine-age resting pulse rate is lower?"

The Physical: "I will demonstrate that the resting pulse rate is the single most important feature of arterial disease. Let's say that the pre-machine average resting pulse rate was sixty and compare it with today's assumed seventy. That would be 14,400 fewer beats in one day, which would add up to 5,256,000 fewer beats in one year."

The Mental: "Why are all these extra beats so important? I never hear the experts talking about the resting pulse rate."

The Physical: "You're right. One of science's fundamental laws and the one that has been seriously over- looked here is 'action-reaction'. This means that for every action there is a reaction. In our example above, five million unnecessary blows are being struck on the fork of an artery in one year. What is the reaction? The reaction is premature damage. Call it a thickening of the arterial wall, call it scarring, call it hardening of the arteries, or call it arteriosclerosis. This condition is caused by an excessive resting pulse rate."

CHAPTER NINE

AEROBICS AND ARTERIOSCLEROSIS

In which slowing that resting pulse rate is discussed.

The Mental: "So, is exercise the answer to this problem?"

The Physical: "Yes, the answer is aerobic exercise. Aerobic exercise strengthens muscles, both the heart and the arteries. In fact, aerobic exercise is the only way this muscle group can be strengthened. An increase in strength means that each stroke is stronger and more efficient and therefore, fewer strokes are necessary. This causes the resting pulse rate to go down."

The Emotional: "This means fewer of those destructive pulsations you were talking about."

The Physical: "Yes, and it's the 'Use it or lose it' law. When the heart and arteries never get exercised they become weaker and less efficient. As the arterial system gets weaker, more beats are required to supply the same amount of blood. This causes the resting pulse rate to rise."

The Mental: "So the most important reason for aerobics is to lower the resting pulse rate?"

The Physical: "That's correct. I once knew 'Elaine', a rather sedentary girl, who began a running program in a physical education class. She ran two miles three days a week. When Elaine entered the class, her resting pulse rate was 82 beats per minute. At the end of the nine week grading period, her resting pulse rate had dropped to 57 beats per minute. This meant that Elaine's heart was beating 36,000 fewer times in a 24-hour period. When we multiply this number by weeks, months, and years, the significance of this approach becomes obvious."

The Emotional: "How should we monitor our resting pulse rate?"

The Physical: "For the most reliable consistency, do your pulse rate check before getting out of bed in the morning. Place three fingers on the outside of your up-turned wrist or on the carotid artery in your neck. Be sure to use fingers and not the thumb. The thumb can provide false pulsations and is less reliable. Count the pulsations for fifteen seconds and multiply by four."

The Emotional: "Wow, the most important health measurement, self-administered, in just fifteen seconds!"

The Mental: "What about the range? What are the highs and lows?"

The Physical: "The range is from the low forties and sometimes lower, to one hundred and sometimes higher."

The Mental: "So what should the resting pulse rate target be?"

The Physical: "Once again, the current average resting pulse rate is somewhere in the seventies. That figure is the result of research conducted during the modern era. Pre-machine average resting pulse rate was much lower but we will never know by how much.

It's just a guess, but probably sixty and under would be a healthy target."

BEATS/MIN	BEATS/DAY	BEATS/MIN	BEATS/DAY
100	144000	69	99360
99	142560	68	97920
98	141120	67	96480
97	139680	66	95040
96	138240	65	93600
95	136800	64	92160
94	135360	63	90720
93	133920	62	89280
92	132480	61	87840
91	131040	60	86400
90	129600	59	84960
89	128160	58	83520
88	126720	57	82080
87	125280	56	80640
86	123840	55	79200
85	122400	54	77760
84	120960	53	76320
83	119520	52	74380
82	118080	51	73440
81	116640	50	72000
80	115200	49	70560
79	113760	48	69180
78	112320	47	67680
77	110880	46	66240
76	109440	45	64800
75	108000	44	63360
74	106560	43	61920
73	105120	42	60480
72	103680	41	59840
71	i02240	40	57690
70	100800		

CHAPTER TEN

OTHER CONDITIONS THAT CHANGE THE RESTING PULSE RATE

We name three villains, smoking, overweight, and stress.

The Mental: "Is aerobic exercise the only way that the resting pulse rate can be altered?"

The Physical: "It's the only way that it can be improved or lowered. However, there are some other problems that cause the resting pulse rate to rise. During the 20th century, smoking was identified as a high-risk behavior for arterial disease. The unrecognized reason is the higher resting pulse rate."

The Mental: "I never hear anything about smoking and the resting pulse rate."

The Physical: "That's because the resting pulse rate has not, until now, been identified as the most significant feature of arterial disease. Smoking interferes with the lung's blood oxygen exchange. This means that the system must beat more times in order to supply the required oxygen. Up goes the resting pulse rate."

The Emotional: "Hey, that explanation really fits."
The Physical: "A possibly more serious negative

effect of smoking is that, generally, those who smoke don't feel like participating in aerobic activities."

The Mental: "Because many smokers don't exercise,

begs the question, is it smoking that's doing the damage or is it the absence of aerobics?"

The Physical: "Next is the overweight dilemma. When people are overweight, their arterial systems must supply a larger volume in the body. Up goes the resting pulse rate. As with the smoker, the overweight individual will find aerobics uncomfortable and something to be avoided. Finally there is stress."

The Emotional: "Hey, wait a minute. Stress is my baby. I'll take this one. Stress is often mentioned as being a contributor to arterial disease. Here, humans have truly put the cart before the horse."

The Mental: "Emotional, you're out of touch."

The Emotional: "For some reason, humans always consider outside-the-body causes first. We blame influences such as relationships, overcrowding, jobs, or traffic."

The Mental: "Certainly you're not going to tell us that these aren't stress creating situations, when we know perfectly well that they are?"

The Physical: Perhaps one of the most important misconceptions centers around the substance known as C-Reactive Protein that measures inflammation within the arterial system, both amount and location.

The Mental: Why haven't we heard about this before?

The Physical: Because inflammation is so prevalent among those tested with no apparent cause, professional interest has waned.

The Emotional: But inflammation is not natural. There has to be a cause. So, what have we learned?

The Physical: Two important facts were exposed

in the research. First, the inflammation interfered with arterial flexibility (hardening of the arteries). Second, the inflammation was greatest where the arteries forked.

The Mental: Somehow, I think you are bringing the resting pulse rate into this.

The Physical: "You're correct. It makes too much sense. I can't resist. Arterial disease does not just suddenly appear. It develops over a lifetime. Using our prior formula, in which our proposed 60 beats per minute, is 5 million annual beats less than todays average 70 beats per minute, let's apply it to a 40-year lifespan. We are now talking about a difference of two hundred million excessive, but aerobically avoidable, lifetime beats pounding on the arterial forks. Which most likely, explains why the higher resting pulse rate is the source of the previously unexplained inflammation."

The Emotional: "Two hundred million extra beats! You've made a believer out of me."

The Physical: "Yes Emotional, we must apply the scientific action-reaction rule. By using that rule we are providing a very logical cause to the identified C-Reactive Protein inflammation. And more important than that, the C-Reactive Protein has identified the arterial forks as having the greatest accumulation of inflammation. The same forks that lie in the direct path of two hundred million extra beats that can only be lowered by aerobic exercise."

The Emotional: "No, Mental I'm not, but I do feel that it's best to start on the inside and work out. It's the rapid internal rhythm of the accelerated resting pulse rate that makes me feel stressful just as the slower internal rhythm of the lower resting pulse rate tends to make me feel more relaxed and in a better position to deal with the out- of-body frustrations."

The Mental: "How can you compare that internal accelerated rhythm to all the other identified causes of stress?"

The Emotional: "Easy. In fact, of all identified causes of stress, the internal rhythm of the resting pulse rate is not only the most important but is also the single contributing factor that the individual actually has some control over."

The Mental: "Isn't it true that many people practice yoga and meditation to relieve stress, and they often claim that they can lower the heart rate?

The Emotional: "These methods are often successful. The lower heart rate, however, will only be created for that particular session, if at all, and not for the full twenty-four hours a day as would be the case with the aerobically lowered resting pulse rate."

The Physical: "Once again we've got it backwards. Instead of saying that stress causes arterial disease, we should say that it is the accelerated resting pulse rate of arterial disease that causes stress."

The Emotional: "Yes, Physical, your aerobic exercise is important when it comes to fighting stress because it slows down that internal rhythm that we are never without. This is the reason that aerobic athletes consistently demonstrate more favorable scores on stress tests."

CHAPTER ELEVEN

HOW HARDENING OF THE ARTERIES AND EXCESSIVE CHOLESTEROL WORK TOGETHER

Understanding arterial disease's deadly partnership.

The Mental: "Well, Physical if hardening of the arteries is caused by an elevated resting pulse rate, why are damaged areas covered with extra-heavy amounts of cholesterol?"

The Physical: "It's really the relationship between arteriosclerosis and atherosclerosis, cholesterol, that is important to understand. Because there is always excessive cholesterol around arteriosclerosis, it is believed that it's the cholesterol that is responsible, actually causing this thickening of the arterial wall. In fact, it's the other way around."

The Mental: "You're like a salmon going up-stream. This is really against current thinking."

The Physical: "Remember that when we talk about controlling excessive cholesterol, the most important change created by aerobics is the expansion and contraction of the artery."

The Mental: "Yes, I remember the natural and constant aerobic fluctuation to the inside wall of the artery that you mentioned; and the disturbance that prevents excessive cholesterol from building up."

The Physical: "Very good, Mental. Arteriosclerosis, excuse me Emotional, hardening of the arteries, caused by an excessive resting pulse rate, means that the affected arterial area, usually the fork, becomes scarred, thickened, and hardened."

The Mental: "Why is it called hardening of the arteries'?"

The Physical: "Because the accelerated resting pulse rate causes damage that results in scarring. This scarred material is bigger and harder and less flexible than normal tissue."

The Mental: "OK, continue."

The Physical: "This condition is serious because where this damage occurs, the artery can no longer expand and contract. The inactivity of the damaged area encourages the build-up of excessive atherosclerosis. It's a combination of the thickening of the arterial wall and the resulting excessive build-up of cholesterol that so dangerously narrows the inside diameter of the artery."

The Mental: "How does this narrowed condition contribute to a heart attack or as you call it, an arterial occlusion?"

The Physical: "The accelerated resting pulse rate scars and thickens the artery at the fork. Excessive cholesterol develops on the inactive area and a combination of these two conditions can completely block the artery.

The Mental: "All this talk about exercise. Isn't it true that early in the 20th century, exercise was thought to be responsible for heart disease? Don't we still hear warnings about exercise today?"

The Physical: "Yes, it's important for inactive humans to enter exercise programs gradually. A typical exercise-induced heart attack would be as follows: A sedentary person suddenly experiences extreme emotion or engages in heavy physical exercise. With this increased activity, arteries that have been inactive suddenly are forced to expand. This causes excessive atherosclerosis to be dislodged from the inside wall of the artery."

The Mental: "Is that dangerous?"

The Physical: "This material travels down the system until it comes to a fork where a combination of hardening of the arteries and excessive cholesterol have dangerously narrowed the inside diameter of the artery. The dislodged material gets stuck in the narrow spot and creates an arterial occlusion."

The Emotional: "How come some heart attack victims survive?"

The Physical: "If it's a minor artery, the individual will probably recover. If it's a major artery, survival will be threatened. It's this reaction within the arterial system of a sedentary person that leads to warnings about beginning exercise programs slowly."

The Emotional: "Along these same lines, the marvelous drug Viagra has been developed to assist my all important sexual behavior."

The Mental: "Oh Emotional, where are you off to now?"

The Emotional: "Hey! usually medical supervision is required. Male humans who have been diagnosed with arterial problems have been warned about using this drug. Viagra not only expands the arteries in the penis, but throughout the rest of the body as well. Arteries of a sedentary individual are unaccustomedly forced to expand. Just as with beginning aerobics, this expansion may dislodge excessive cholesterol from the inner wall of the artery."

The Mental: "Well, to sum up, Physical, that explains excessive cholesterol or atherosclerosis and arteriosclerosis or hardening of the arteries and how they work together. Now explain your third factor in arterial disease, collateral circulation."

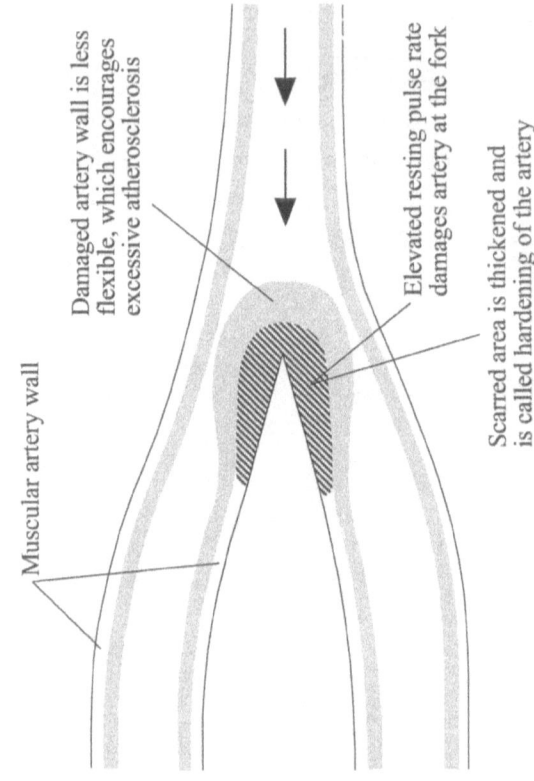

HARDENING OF THE ARTERY

Muscular artery wall

Damaged artery wall is less flexible, which encourages excessive atherosclerosis

Elevated resting pulse rate damages artery at the fork

Scarred area is thickened and is called hardening of the artery or artereosclerosis

CHAPTER TWELVE

COLLATERAL CIRCULATION

Maximum system efficiency.

The Physical: "Collateral circulation refers to how many of the available arteries are being used. Let's say that we have two cell masses, one belonging to an athlete and one belonging to a sedentary person. Let's further say that each cell mass has five tiny arteries supplying it. Because for the sedentary person the demand on the cell mass is very low, one artery gets the job done and the other four arteries are in a latent state, 'present but not being used'."

The Mental: "How does aerobics come into play here?"

The Physical: "Aerobics forces all available arteries to be used. Because of our athlete's aerobic exercise, increased demand forces all five arteries that supply that cell mass to function. If the artery supplying the sedentary cell mass should fail, that cell mass would be in trouble. If one of the five arteries to our athlete's cell mass should fail, there would be a healthy one alongside to take up the slack."

The Mental: "Does collateral circulation happen all over the body?"

The Physical: "Yes, but weak collateral circulation usually occurs at the ends, furthest from the heart. This is the distal end of the arterial system, where blood is distributed through smaller vessels by the pressure created by the contractions closer to the heart. The closer the arteries are to the source of the pulsations, the greater the effects on arteriosclerosis and the resulting build-up of cholesterol. As the blood moves away from the heart and the major arteries, the pulsations become weaker. It's at this point that collateral circulation's many tiny arteries that furnish blood to capillaries are filled with blood from the pressure established closer to the center of the system. Extremities sometimes have weak circulation because they are far from the heart. A weak arterial system has difficulty delivering blood to the extremities."

The Mental: "Are there warning signs with this problem?"

The Physical: "Cooled skin temperatures and numbness in the hands and feet are often clues to weak collateral circulation. The head isn't usually considered to be an extremity but it should be."

The Mental: "Why is that? The head isn't that far from the heart."

The Physical: "It's not because it's far from the heart, but because the blood to it defies gravity. The arterial system works hard to deliver blood up to the head and your brain. Sometimes humans will rise up too quickly and experience dizziness. This can be a sign of weak collateral circulation."

The Mental: "Are you saying that this collateral circulation thing could influence my brain?"

The Physical: "Yes, weak collateral circulation has a major impact on stroke. Your brain, the most important feature of your nervous system, is more threatened by stroke than by any other difficulty."

The Mental: "I thought stroke was a different problem."

The Physical: "That's understandable. Throughout the 20th century and up to the present, stroke has been placed in a category by itself. Most strokes occur when the arterial system can't supply blood to the brain or parts of the brain. That ischemic stroke we talked about earlier is clearly the result of arterial disease. We need only to imagine that the cell masses that we used as examples before are cell masses in your brain."

The Emotional: "Yeah, Mental, and what if it was the memory center of your brain that was experiencing this weak collateral circulation?"

The Mental: "What do you mean?"

The Emotional: "Well isn't the increasingly inactive technological society, you created, becoming more and more concerned about loss of memory?"

The Mental: "Don't be silly."

The Emotional: "I'm not being silly. It makes perfect sense. We established that these arterial problems were degenerative. We know that as humans age they become less active. Once again we can refer to the 'Use it or lose it' law. As less and less demand is placed on the arterial system, collateral circulation will certainly withdraw. Mental, it seems reasonable to me that dementia or any number of problems could occur because of weak collateral circulation to your all-important brain."

The Physical: "Any way you look at it, aerobic exercise is the only way to strengthen and maintain strong collateral circulation. It forces all available arteries to be used."

The Mental: "We hear so much about blood pressure, does that fit in here?"

The Physical: "Like the resting pulse rate, high blood pressure or hypertension, as it's often called, is a relatively new body measurement. In many respects, it also remains a mystery. It makes sense, however, that clogged, narrowed, and inactive arteries should be the first consideration. Weakened arterial muscle and clogged arteries combined with the use of fewer arteries means that the system must beat more rapidly and apply more pressure to those arteries still functioning."

The Mental: "What's this business about growing new arteries?"

The Physical: "I'm not sure, but it makes sense that it could be the result of observing inactive individuals as they increase their exercise level. Aerobic exercise forces all available arteries to be used. That physical demand makes latent arteries active participants in the circulatory process."

The Emotional: "It seems to me that the terms collateral circulation and hypertension are interchangeable."

The Physical: "Not really. The condition of collateral circulation would have to be the most important factor when considering blood pressure test results. A condition that can only be improved with aerobic exercise."

The Mental: "My observations have medicine as the most frequently recommended remedy for hypertension."

The Physical: "That's correct. However, medicine represents temporary outside relief, and may have to be administered for very long periods or perhaps a lifetime."

The Mental: "I hear that drugs are often accompanied by negative side effects."

The Physical: "Yes. Aerobic exercise is the only way to create and maintain natural and healthy collateral circulation."

The Emotional: "I like that. Solving the problem from the inside out."

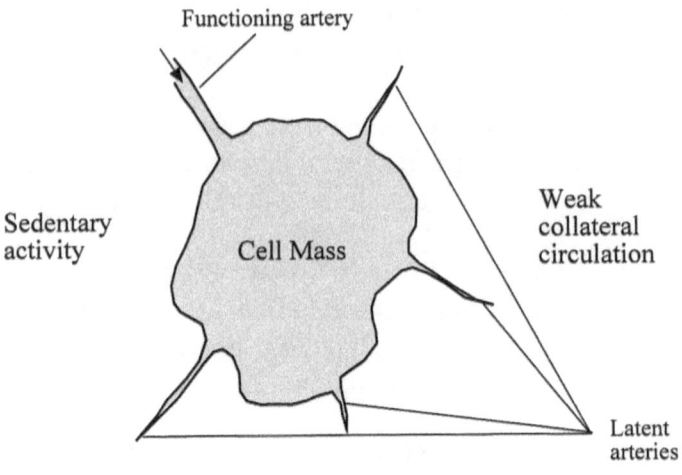

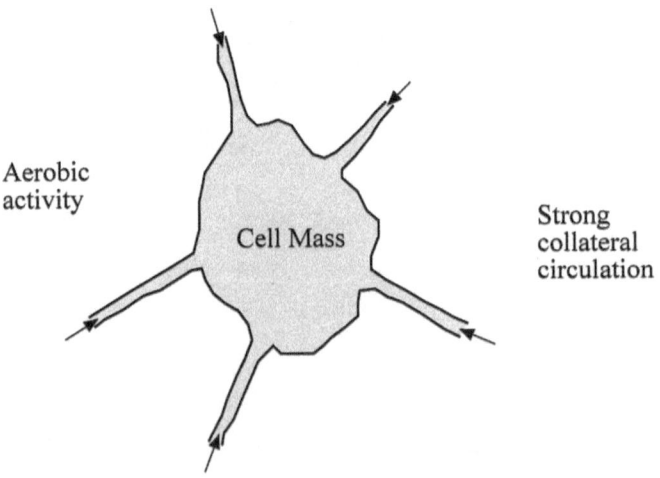

COLLATERAL CIRCULATION

CHAPTER THIRTEEN

MORE MISCONCEPTIONS

In which we are sidetracked along the way.

The Physical: "Because we're talking about a weakened muscle system, exercise should be our number one priority when it comes to prevention and treatment."

The Emotional: "This isn't the case. Generally, arterial difficulties are treated with diet and medicine first."

The Physical: "Mental, you were right when you said that most often irregular blood pressure is treated with medicine. There isn't now, nor is it likely that there ever will be, a medicine that can permanently improve collateral circulation. This can only be achieved with aerobic exercise. It's the same aerobic activity that was commonplace, before your technology, throughout our entire evolutionary past."

The Mental: "Quit beating up on my technology. Are there other 20th century misconceptions?"

The Physical: "During the early part of the 20th century, heart disease was thought to be almost exclusively a male affliction. This is because the machine took all the heavy aerobic-type labor out of most industries. Industrial heavy labor during the early part of the century, was done by a predominantly male work force. During this period, the change in activity levels was much greater for males than for females. By the end of the 20th century, modern technology had become all-encompassing, and the incidence of female arterial disease had caught up with that of the male."

The Emotional: "And then there's that exercise mix- up."

The Physical: "Yes, in the first half of the twentieth century, heart attacks occurred most often when individuals were engaged in exercise. This observation resulted in patients being bed-ridden and a preventative warning was issued to the public at large that strenuous activities should be avoided."

The Emotional: "I can remember the comments about staying off Cardiac Hill."

The Physical: "Certainly exercise may trigger arterial disease but only after long periods of inactivity. Here at the beginning of the 21st century, our ideas about exercise are back on the right track, but they still play second fiddle to diet in terms of preventative importance."

The Mental: "I always feel like my technology is being blamed for a change in diet."

The Physical: "We really don't have to be concerned about modern technology's impact on our diet. As a species, we humans have proved we can survive nicely on a wide range of diets from total meat eating to total vegetarianism. Technology has had a relatively small impact on human diet except to make food more available and to provide a greater variety."

The Mental: "You continue to belittle the importance of diet."

The Physical: "That's not true. It's simply a matter of priorities. Diet is important but not as important as aerobic exercise, especially when it comes to arterial disease. It's our exercise level that has been tremendously altered or eliminated by your third shock."

The Mental: "Most wouldn't agree."

The Physical: "Mental, your technology has changed diet in that all of the physical activity required to produce it has been lost. The high-tech human animal is the only creature known that can avoid personal production or acquisition of its own food supply. By using the machine, a very few can produce enough for very many."

The Emotional: "I can remember that during the sixties of the 20th century there was an article in which someone had conducted a study showing that significant numbers of people were having heart attacks during the night while they were sleeping."

The Physical: "People having heart attacks while they are at complete rest is possible but rare."

The Emotional: "I agree and have a theory about that. For inactive individuals, having infrequent sex could be a life-threatening experience. This is the most logical explanation for so many individuals having heart attacks while at reported complete rest. Rather than face an embarrassing revelation, it was easier for the surviving partner, usually a woman, to say that her partner had passed away in his sleep."

CHAPTER FOURTEEN

FEELING GOOD AND AEROBICS

The 'Emotion' talks about getting high.

The Mental: "Is sex all you ever think about?"

The Emotional: "No but I must admit that, for me, it's a biggie. In fact, research tells us that people who are physically fit experience sex more often and with more enjoyment."

The Mental: "Now there's a real selling point."

The Emotional: "Listen, before you guys interrupted me, I was talking about exercise and feeling good. During the seventies of the last century the industrial complex began spending mega-bucks installing physical fitness facilities for their employees."

The Physical: "That's true."

The Emotional: "They didn't do this out of the kindness of their heart, no pun intended, but rather because extensive insurance research pointed out that people who are physically fit feel better about themselves. People who feel better about themselves are more productive. The pay-off for industry was increased employee productivity."

The Mental: "I remember that. In fact, many industries today encourage their employees to be active."

The Emotional: "When people who are constantly involved in aerobics are asked why they do it, the overwhelming answer is not about arterial health, but rather that it makes them feel good."

The Physical: "The reason being, that an aerobic person has placed him or her self in balance with a naturally active past. If we bring balance to the arterial system, the system that extends to every part of the body, we will surely realize mental and emotional benefits."

The Emotional: "Remember, it's impossible to separate us. The physical, the mental, and the emotional. We are all one."

The Mental: "Yes, but today's society seems to want to divide us."

The Physical: "There are a few fundamental body functions that should occur on a daily basis. We should consume food, we should exercise, we should rest, and we should eliminate. It's this elimination function that receives too little attention."

The Mental: "Many physicians claim that daily or semi-daily elimination is not necessary."

The Physical: "And most of us do not, so those physicians have made a reasonable assumption."

The Emotional: "That is a good example of the scientific world forming an opinion because of a fact derived from studying an inactive society. Also, a great deal of scientific information is derived from studying rats and other animals whose activity levels have been heavily restricted inside laboratories."

The Physical: "There's much more time spent being concerned about what goes into our bodies than there is time spent worrying about how it comes out. People who are sedentary usually do not eliminate on a daily schedule. They may go two, three, four, and not uncommonly more days without defecating."

The Emotional: "This means that those individuals are storing toxic waste material for unreasonable periods of time. How can an individual feel good when that kind of chemical imbalance exists?"

The Mental: "This is a problem that can be solved with diet including lots of fruits and vegetables. Not only that, but the modern medicine cabinet is loaded with numerous medicines that relieve constipation."

The Physical: "It's true, those are solutions. On the other hand, another one of the beautiful results of aerobic exercise is regularity. It would be very difficult to find an aerobic athlete who doesn't eliminate on a daily basis. The exercise changes the metabolism and there's a more natural demand for more energy, and increased production of waste. There's a more balanced exchange."

The Mental: "Yeah, but my solution of using diet and drugs is a lot easier than aerobic exercise."

The Emotional: "Well it makes sense to me that the aerobic solution should be applied, because it positively affects so many other areas. Once again, it's treating the problem from the inside out."

The Mental: "Well what about drugs? Don't people take drugs in order to feel good?"

The Physical: "Yes of course. The problem here is that people who do drugs don't feel like exercising."

The Mental: "Well, if the idea is to feel good then why not take drugs? It's a lot easier."

The Emotional: "Much of human expression is a combination of positive and negative addictions. The secret here is to keep the positive habits ahead of the negative."

The Mental: "How can you tell the difference between the two?"

The Emotional: "Well I once heard that a negative addiction feels good while it's happening, feels terrible right afterwards, and generally detracts from an individual's overall life experience. Alcohol is a beautiful example. On the other hand, positive addiction feels uncomfortable or challenging while it's happening; it feels terrific when it's over; and it generally makes a contribution to the individual's overall life experience. Certainly, consistent exercising is a wonderful example of a positive addiction."

The Mental: "Many experts are saying that alcoholism is not an addiction, but that it's a disease and a disease encouraged by genetics."

The Emotional: "I don't believe that drugs are a disease. It's easy to establish a habit around a substance that produces pleasure. Habit is a part of all animal life. An individual may be prone to stronger or weaker habitual activity because of genetics but not to the substance or behavior itself. Offenders must create a habit that denies the urge for the substance, each time it arises. In so doing, they use the power of the positive habit to counteract the power of the negative habit."

The Mental: "That's all well and good but, Emotional, sometimes you have a way of making complicated issues sound too simple."

The Emotional: "No, it's not simple or easy but the ultimate answer is creating a positive habit that denies the negative habit. A denial addiction."

The Mental: "What about the overeating habit? Total denial isn't possible."

The Emotional: "You're right, it's a much more challenging form of habit reversal."

The Physical: "Why is the overeating habit more difficult than others?"

The Emotional: "Most other negative habits like drugs, aren't a necessary part of life and therefore total denial or complete separation can be practiced. Food, on the other hand, is a required pleasure."

The Physical: "So the problem can't be avoided and total separation can't be achieved."

The Emotional: "That's correct."

The Physical: "So what's the solution?"

The Emotional: "The answer is the more difficult partial denial. When overeating is the problem, the victim must find a way to express self-denial in the midst of a highly pleasurable experience. The victim must apply partial denial at the second helping or whatever is perceived to be 'over the line'. Partial denial is the hardest challenge because it's continuous."

The Physical: "Well, this hi-tech society has reduced the activity level and increased the food supply so that its citizens are generally overweight."

CHAPTER FIFTEEN

AEROBICS AND FAT

The 'Physical' talks about aerobics, the fat burner.

The Mental: "When the experts talk about losing weight, they usually suggest eating less and exercising. How does exercise fit in?"

The Physical: "Metabolism is the chemical reaction in the cell that creates energy for needed activities. Each cell in the body has fat burning enzymes and fat storing enzymes. This is because, for all the time preceding modern technology, we went from feast to famine."

The Emotional: "There's no famine in our nation."

The Physical: "The human body and the bodies of other animals have evolved with fat storing enzymes so that they can store fat or food for the lean times. These enzymes are trained by us. For the athlete, the fat burning enzymes are being trained. This is because the fat is being used to fuel the activity."

The Mental: "What about the sedentary person?"

The Physical: "The inactive person is also training enzymes, but instead of training fat burning enzymes they are training their fat storing enzymes. Like anything else in nature, the more something is repeated the stronger it becomes. The more we train either fat burning or fat storing enzymes, the better they get at performing their task."

The Mental: "I suppose your aerobic exercise is the answer here as well."

The Physical: "Yes, the absolutely best training program for fat burning enzymes is aerobic exercise. The best training program for fat storing enzymes is doing nothing. Mental, in your modern society, watching television is an excellent way to develop fat storing enzymes."

The Mental: "Does this change in the burning process occur only during the activity period?"

The Physical: "No, the change in metabolism is for the entire twenty-four-hour period and not just for the exercise session. The active individual is burning more calories while driving the car, doing the dishes, and sleeping at night.

The Emotional: "I can't tell you how much stress time I spend being concerned over the hundreds of diets that are invented each year. I go absolutely nuts at the beginning of each year over broken resolutions. I conclude that this is unnecessary anxiety when it's been proven that the 'bottom line' is to eat less and exercise more."

The Physical: "Aerobics are effective because usually the large leg muscles are involved and they create a large demand. For best results, the upper body skeletal muscles should be included in the exercise plan as well."

The Emotional: "When we consider Mental's technological changes, Physical, you're lucky. You've been able to identify a major change in individual behavior and provide us with a solution. I, also, am able to observe some fundamental deviations in our social structure created by technology. However, because the problem is more complicated when extended to more than one individual, solutions are not currently apparent."

The Mental: "I was hoping we could avoid the social stuff. My technology is really taking a beating."

The Physical: "You needn't worry. Human technology will always continue to survive and thrive. It's just interesting and important to observe changes in fundamental behavior."

The Mental: "What are you calling fundamental behavior? Are your aerobics fundamental?"

The Physical: "Of course. It's all those things that occurred consistently prior to your modern technology. I'm sure there are many others besides activity level."

The Mental: "Oh yeah, like what?"

The Physical: "Well, one example might be that because of your technology, humans have gone from being an outdoor animal to being an indoor animal."

The Mental: "What's the big deal about that?"

The Physical: "I have no idea. It just seems like an example of a fundamental change."

The Emotional: "You guys are going on about nothing and just trying to distract me from my social concerns."

The Mental: "OK, Emotional, you go."

CHAPTER SIXTEEN

TECHNOLOGY AND THE FAMILY

The 'Emotional' explains how technology has ripped
some long standing social fabric.

The Emotional: "I believe our living changes
coming from eliminating human participation in food
acquisition and production have been huge. Not just,
as The Physical pointed out, because of the reduction
in activity, but even more important because it has
been the foundation for human interconnectedness."

The Mental: "What makes you think that?"

The Emotional: "It's one of two main reasons
humans have become group animals. First, because
the family worked together for producing and sharing
food and second, the extremely long nurturing period
for young humans requires teamwork."

The Mental: "Certainly humans can survive on
their own."

The Emotional: "In your modern world yes, an
adult can survive on his or her own. With the human
species, however, the young are totally dependent on
some form of parenting for the first five to ten years of
their lives and usually longer. It's this early
dependency that creates the adult team. For most of
us, this teamwork has always centered around food.
Mental your technology has removed the biggest
reason for human bonding."

The Mental: "I wish you guys would stop being such crybabies. Because of me, those humans living in developed areas don't have to worry all day about producing their own food. They can kick back and take it easy. Instead of hunting and gathering, growing, or herding their own food, they can purchase it."

The Emotional: "The change has been so swift and complete that we humans fail to recognize the interpersonal responsibilities and social skills that the earlier feeding pattern demanded."

The Mental: "Getting rid of it frees up large chunks of time with which people can fantasize about other areas of existence. My technology has relieved humans of their most significantly demanding and time-consuming animal behavior, getting fed."

The Emotional: "Yes, Mental, I understand the apparent advantages. However, there are some important family and community changes that worry me. Hunting and gathering dominated the human feeding pattern for most of the human past."

The Mental: "Yes, with hunting being the most important."

The Emotional: "No, that may not be true. There was an anthropologist who chose to reverse the description of this period from "hunter gatherer" to "gatherer hunter". He explained that hunters failed most of the time whereas gatherers were more consistent suppliers of food, and most responsible for human survival."

The Mental: "I must admit that the hunter has fallen on hard times."

The Emotional: "In gathering and hunting cultures and even through most of the agriculture period, the successful hunter was the pillar of the community. Your third shock has made hunting obsolete."

The Physical: "Yes, killing wild animals has become sport and, for many, very unpopular."

The Emotional: "At the end of the 20th century, the hunter was considered the low-life and about to get kicked off the bottom rung of the social ladder."

The Mental: "Well, hunting has simply become unnecessary."

The Emotional: "This could have an important impact on young males. Because of the long period of early human dependency, there is a powerful drive in all young humans to achieve independent adulthood."

The Mental: "That's always been true."

The Emotional: "Throughout history, most societies had 'Rites of Passage' for young males, a social ceremony to move the male from adolescence into adulthood."

The Physical: "And hunting was often that vehicle."

The Emotional: "There were others. The successful warrior for instance, but the most common form of Rite of Passage was the young hunter's first hunting kill and its opportunity to provide food for the group. Mental, in your modern world there are no group survival contributions or ceremonies to define male adulthood."

The Mental: "What about female adulthood?

The Emotional: "The adulthood problem for females was solved through menstruation and or childbearing. Could it be that today's gang mentality for young males is an ugly substitute for the Rites of Passage?"

The Mental: "Now my all-important technology is being held responsible for young male violence. Come on Emotional, Get a grip. You spend too much time worrying about all those leftover behaviors from all that primitive time. Get with the modern world."

The Physical: "The human gene pool inherits behavior most of all from that primitive time."

The Emotional: "No, Mental, I'm not through. You know how important sexuality is to me. I think you'll agree that during the 20th century a serious degeneration of the family structure occurred. At the beginning of the 20th century, divorce was relatively rare and usually accompanied by social condemnation."

The Physical: "By coincidence, at the beginning of the 20th century most humans were still involved in food raising and producing."

The Emotional: "At the conclusion of the century, divorce and separation were not only socially acceptable, but were ending well over fifty percent of all marriages."

The Mental: "First, I'm responsible for weak arterial muscle and then young male confusion and now I'm the reason for accelerated divorce rates."

The Emotional: "Yes Mental, your modern world is a major contributor. Before the machine age, males and females labored in separate work groups."

The Physical: "That's correct. Because they are bigger and stronger, males did the heavy work, usually hunting or in the field, and females did the jobs of gathering or working near the home."

The Emotional: "Large portions of time spent in separate work groups created minimal sexual exposure and stimulation. Mechanizing in your modern machine age meant that the females could push the buttons as well as the males, so that both could work side-by-side in the same work force. Advanced technology meant that for the first time in the history of our species, males and females could labor in the same survival groups. Continuous exposure meant increased male-female sexual stimulation."

The Mental: "OK, that makes sense."

The Emotional: "The other altered factor in this formula deals with social control of sexual behavior. For all the time before the machine age most humans lived in family groups or small rural communities. One small town syndrome is that everyone knows what everyone else is doing."

The Mental: "Isn't that still true?"

The Emotional: "Your high-tech industrialism drew large numbers of humans to the cities and created huge urban living conditions. Extracurricular sexual behavior often goes unnoticed in large city communities."

The Mental: "That's true, I never thought of that before."

The Emotional: "So, prior to modern technology, males and females worked in separate work forces, which meant much less sexual stimulation; and they lived in small communities, which meant that when they were together there was maximum social control.

Since the spread of your modern technology, males and females work in the same work force, which means maximum sexual stimulation; and because they live together in such large numbers there is minimum social control."

The Physical: "That's very interesting Emotional. I've been so busy worrying about how technology has reduced human activity levels, I never stopped to consider the social ramifications."

The Emotional: "Yes, it's my view that this high-tech environment with it's distracting sexual reality combined with the elimination of the inter-personal survival responsibilities required in dealing with the previous feeding pattern are major contributors to the 20th century's degenerative family structure."

The Mental: "That's an interesting theory and you are probably right, but so what? There's no going back and those times are gone forever. Once again it's adaptability that will most contribute to human survival. All the changes of the 20th century will be dwarfed by the changes that will occur in the 21st. We must concentrate on the future."

The Physical: "You're right, there is no going back. However, we are clearly products of all of our past. The more we understand about our past, the better off we are when it comes to making decisions about the present and the future. Humans will be better at adapting."

CHAPTER SEVENTEEN

HOW MUCH AEROBICS?

Here the conversation turns to activities, duration and frequency.

The Mental: "Well, how much of this aerobic exercise should be happening and how often should it occur?"

The Physical: "That's a difficult question, because it's different for each individual."

The Emotional: "There must be some aerobic fundamentals that we could use as a guide."

The Physical: "Yes, and frequency is one of those fundamentals. Many athletes prefer to exercise daily."

The Emotional: "I don't know if I can get into that routine."

The Physical: "Yes, those athletes believe that aerobic exercise is one of life's daily health events. Most experts agree that the minimum should be three days a week."

The Emotional: "I hear some people say they realize the important health benefits of exercising, but just don't have the time."

The Physical: "I always find that to be an interesting reaction since we're talking about the single best way to add years of active enjoyable life."

The Emotional: "O well, life is full of priorities."

The Mental: "What aerobic activities are best?"

The Physical: "Activities that involve the legs are important because they have large muscles and exercising them creates the big increase in demand that triggers the aerobic expression."

The Mental: "Obviously, the participants' interest and available facilities are important considerations."

The Physical: "Yes. Distance swimming would be the single best overall body exercise, but swimming facilities may not be available to everyone. Running, hiking, and cycling are the most popular."

The Mental: "I hear that the jarring involved in running leads to injuries."

The Physical: "Running may not be for everyone. Certainly, running on a soft surface can help."

The Emotional: "What about walking? It's very popular."

The Physical: "Walking is a wonderful activity used by many.

This is a good time to say a little about another aerobic fundamental, exertion."

The Mental: "What do you mean by exertion?"

The Physical: "Exertion represents the modest increase in activity level required in order to strengthen arterial muscle. Remember that the primary goal of aerobic exercise is to strengthen arterial muscle. Doing this lowers the resting pulse rate."

The Emotional: "Is that 'exertion' what they mean when they say, 'No pain no gain'?"

The Physical: "I'm not sure that exertion should be called pain, but it's for the total body, and sometimes an uncomfortable, challenge."

The Mental: "How about those people who say that exertion or being uncomfortable isn't necessary during exercise."

The Physical: "That's what I call 'maintenance' and there's nothing wrong with that. Something is better than nothing. However, moderate exertion should be the goal; it will result in an increase in strength."

The Emotional: "How can we recognize 'exertion'?"

The Physical: "As I mentioned earlier, there should be 15 to 20 minutes or more of oxygen debt activity that results in mild perspiration."

The Mental: "You haven't mentioned stretching. There are lots of experts and books that concentrate on the importance of stretching for all forms of exercise."

The Physical: "You're right. Stretching is important before and after all exercise."

The Emotional: "Hey, we're talking about the arterial muscles here. I certainly don't see how we're going to stretch that system."

The Physical: "We solve that problem by utilizing the most important aerobic fundamental of all."

The Mental: "What's that?"

The Physical: "Start out slowly."

The Mental: "Start out slowly?"

The Physical: "Yes. Start out slowly and then build gradually to your exertion level. It's a big transition for the body to move from complete rest to exertion. This change is the most challenging part of aerobic exercise. Moving through this transitional phase too quickly can be very uncomfortable and ruin the entire aerobic experience. By moving forward slowly, you will feel much stronger at the exertion level."

The Emotional: "I wonder if that's what people mean when they say that they 'Caught their second wind'. Is that feeling strong at the exertion level?"

The Physical: "Could be."

The Mental: "I'm concerned about over-doing. How can we tell the difference between exertion and over-exertion?"

The Physical: "That's a good question. Fortunately, some of your technology helps give us the answer. There's a wonderful aerobics tool known as the heart monitor. It's an un-incumbering device worn by an exerciser that records the resting pulse rate and the exercising pulse rate; and, most importantly, establishes a predetermined exercise target zone."

The Mental: "That sounds great."

The Physical: "Yes, and it also allows the participant to check recovery time."

The Mental: "What's recovery time? Why is it important?"

The Physical: "It's how long it takes the arterial system to go from exercise pulse rate to resting pulse rate. As you become stronger, you'll take less time for recovery."

The Mental: All this aerobic heavy breathing, should it be through the nose or the mouth?"

The Physical: "Whatever's most comfortable for you. If you're in a state of exertion it's likely that both your nose and your mouth will be anxious to participate. There is, however, a two minute breathing exercise that can be beneficial."

The Mental: "What's that?"

The Physical: "It's called 'forced air breathing'. The working cells of the lungs are called alveoli and are responsible for transfering oxygen from the lungs to the blood. For the first few minutes following the aerobic workout, the lungs are still in oxygen debt but on their way to recovery. The athletes deprive their lungs of oxygen by holding their breath for extended intervals. This forces the alveoli to work hard in order to utilize the reduced available oxygen."

The Emotional: "Doesn't the aerobic workout itself contribute to alveoli function?"

The Physical: "Certainly, but we've worked hard to exercising, and now we have this special two to three minute period following that activity, when we can concentrate on those alveoli and help them to become stronger and more efficient."

The Emotional: "Listen, Physical. You missed, what for me, is a very important aerobic fundamental."

The Physical: "Really, which one is that?"

The Emotional: "Consistency. This is my biggest problem with this exercise business. I have trouble maintaining consistency. I seem to be good at making excuses. I'm in a time crunch, the weather is bad, I don't feel like exercising, and on it goes."

The Physical: "Well, I hope our conversation about the important positive effects that aerobic exercise has on the arterial system will help to motivate us all to bring more consistency to our exercise regimen."

CHAPTER EIGHTEEN

CONCLUSION

The Mental: "Well, perhaps you guys would like to summarize our conversation. I think it's interesting that most of our discussion centered around how a weakened arterial system impacted of itself. I wonder how many other health problems are the result of an early degenerative and out-of-balance supply system? The actual health of the lungs weren't even mentioned, and they are a major player when it comes to aerobics."

The Physical: "I'll go first. Wrongly believing that diet is responsible for excessive cholesterol, and that excessive cholesterol is responsible for excessive arteriosclerosis, has sent us into a diet frenzy. The current social consciousness about preventing and treating arterial disease is that it should be done through diet, with exercise playing a support role. This is like saying that the fuel is more important than the machine. Obviously, it should be the other way around. The post-machine-age human body isn't starving for food, it's starving for activity. We are not what we eat, rather we are what we do. Nothing happens in our lives without muscle involvement, and all muscle obeys the 'Use it or lose it' law.

There's no diet that can cause arteries to expand and contract, disturbing the inner wall and making accumulating of excessive cholesterol very difficult.

Only aerobic exercise can do this. The same aerobics that have been occurring naturally and consistently for all of human time. There's no diet that will significantly lower the resting pulse rate, which in turn reduces hardening of the arteries. Only aerobic exercise can strengthen arterial muscle, which in turn does lower that resting pulse rate. Finally, there's no diet in the world that can force all available arteries to be used, which leads to strong collateral circulation. This can only be done with aerobics."

The Emotional: "All of that aerobic activity slows down my internal resting rhythm, makes me feel more relaxed, and give me emotional strength to cope with outside stresses.

Mostly, it comes down to a matter of priorities. Ask a room full of people to raise their hands if they had brushed their teeth today, and most would raise their hands. Even some of those who did not brush their teeth would raise their hands because we have created a positive social consciousness about taking care of and maintaining that body system. If we ask the same group to raise their hands if they had given any thought to the welfare of their arteries, we would get very different results and from many blank looks. This is an example of mixed-up priorities. If our teeth fall out of our head, we can still survive. If, on the other hand, we develop premature arterial disease, we are now talking about a life-threatening condition. We must find a way to straighten out our priorities so that our muscular arterial system, the system that must supply everything else and the system most threatened, becomes number one.

Earlier I said that my feelings are very important, but depend on our ability to work together. We can't be separated. Physical, if we can all find a way to work together, I'm sure I can give your smile muscles a real workout."

The Mental: "As I claimed before, it is my ability to adapt that most contributes to human survival. You guys have convinced me that the most important health adaptation for now and the future will be consistent aerobic exercise."

THE END

ABOUT THE AUTHOR

Ron Portal is retired after thirty-seven years of teaching physical education in the San Jose Unified School District in California.

Portal says that his career was most influenced by a thirty-five year old heart specialist who was the keynote speaker at a physical education conference in 1961. The doctor provided his audience with a detailed explanation of the effects that aerobic exercise has on the arterial system. The most interesting information he provided was that aerobic exercise lowers the resting pulse rate and that it is the elevated resting pulse rate that causes hardening of the arteries and not cholesterol. Shortly after that presentation, the young doctor unexpectedly died of a brain tumor and his revolutionary ideas about the influence of aerobic exercise were forgotten.

Portal observed that though out the 20th century increased research continued to strongly support the doctor's views about aerobic exercise and improved arterial profiles. Unfortunately the effects were not understood and attempts at an explanation resulted in blind speculation (B.S.).

Frustrated because the current general belief has cholesterol as the villain and diet as the most important preventive feature of arterial disease, Portal became convinced it is time for a change in priorities and there is a need for *Aerobics, The Invisible Advantage*.